TRANSIENT ISCHEMIC ATTACKS

EXPLORING THE WORLD OF TIAs

DR. AHMED .R

Contents

CHAPTER ONE

TIA DEFINITION

Similar symptoms to those of a stroke are produced by transient ischemic attacks (TIAs), which typically persist for a few minutes and do not result in permanent damage.

A transient ischemic attack, often referred to as a ministroke, could be an alert. A stroke will eventually occur in around 1 in 3 persons who experience transient ischemic attacks, with about half of those strokes happening within a year after the transient ischemic attack.

A transient ischemic attack can alert one to the possibility of an approaching stroke and present a chance to take preventative action.

Symptoms

Attacks of transient ischemia often last a few minutes. The majority of symptoms and indicators go away after an hour. Similar to the initial stages of a stroke, transient ischemic attacks (TIAs) can cause sudden start of:

feeling weak, numb, or paralyzed in your arm, leg, or face; usually on one side of the body

speech that is slurred or garbled, or trouble comprehending others

double vision or blindness in one or both eyes

feeling lightheaded or uncoordinated

Depending on which part of the brain is affected, you may experience repeated signs and symptoms from many TIAs.

When to visit a physician

If you believe you may have experienced a transient ischemic attack, get medical help right once. You may be able to prevent a stroke by promptly evaluating and identifying diseases that may be treated.

Reasons

The causes of a transient ischemic attack and ischemic stroke, the most prevalent kind of stroke, are identical. A clot stops part of your brain's blood supply during an ischemic stroke. Unlike a stroke, a transient ischemic attack causes a temporary blockage without causing long-term harm.

The underlying cause of a transient ischemic attack (TIA) is frequently atherosclerosis, or the accumulation of plaques, which are fatty deposits containing cholesterol in an artery or one of its branches that provides your brain with oxygen and nutrition.

A clot may form or the blood flow through an artery may be reduced by a plaque. A transient ischemic attack (TIA) can also be brought on by a blood clot that travels to an artery supplying your brain from another area of your body, usually your heart.

RISK ELEMENTS

It is not possible to modify certain risk factors for transient ischemic attack and stroke. Others are under your authority.

Risk variables that are unchangeable

The following are unchangeable risk factors for stroke and transient ischemic attack. However, being aware of your risk can spur you to alter your way of life in order to lower other hazards.

background in the family. If there is a history of transient ischaemia or stroke in your family, you may be at higher risk.

Years old. As you age, your risk increases; this is particularly true after age 55.

Sexual. Though women account for over half of stroke deaths, men are somewhat more likely to experience TIAs and strokes.

previous brief ischemic episode. You are ten times more likely to have a stroke if you have experienced one or more TIAs.

sickle cell illness. Stroke is a common side effect of sickle cell anemia, another name for this hereditary illness. Blood vessels with a sickle form tend to clog arteries and carry less oxygen, which reduces blood flow to the brain.

Race. Black people have a higher risk of stroke death in part due to their higher rates of diabetes and high blood pressure.

There are several factors that can be controlled or treated to lower your risk of stroke, such as specific medical problems and lifestyle decisions. Although having one or more of these risk factors doesn't guarantee a stroke, having two or more of them raises your risk significantly.

ailments

elevated blood pressure. When blood pressure readings exceed 110/75 millimeters of mercury (mm Hg), there is an increased risk of stroke. Depending on your age, if you have diabetes, and other variables, your doctor will work with you to determine a target blood pressure.

elevated cholesterol. Reducing your intake of cholesterol and fat particularly saturated and trans fats may help your arteries become less plaque-filled. Your doctor might recommend a statin or another kind of cholesterol-lowering medicine if dietary modifications aren't enough to get your cholesterol under control.

heart-related conditions. Heart failure, a cardiac defect, an infection, or an irregular heart rhythm are examples of this.

Carotid artery dysfunction. Your neck's blood arteries that supply your brain stop up.

vascular disease of the peripheral (PAD). Blood clots form in the blood vessels supplying your arms and legs.

CHAPTER TWO

Diabetes. Diabetes accelerates and worsens atherosclerosis, or the narrowing of the arteries brought on by the buildup of fatty deposits.

elevated homocysteine levels. Your arteries may harden and scar as a result of elevated levels of this amino acid in your blood, which increases the risk of clots.

surplus weight. Risk factors include having a waist circumference larger than 35 inches (89 centimeters) for women or 40 inches (102 centimeters) for males, as well as having a body mass index of 25 or above.

smoking of cigarettes. Smoking boosts blood pressure, increases the risk of blood clots, and causes cholesterol-containing fatty deposits to form in your arteries, a condition known as atherosclerosis.

Absence of physical exercise. Almost every day, 30 minutes of moderate-intensity exercise lowers risk.

inadequate diet. Particularly, eating excessive amounts of fat and salt raises your risk of TIA and stroke.

Heavy drinking. If you do drink, try to keep your intake to no more than two drinks for men and one drink for women every day.

usage of illegal substances. Steer clear of illicit narcotics like cocaine.

using birth control tablets. See your doctor about how hormone therapy may impact your risk of stroke and transient ischemic attack (TIA).

Getting Ready for Your Consultation

Although TIAs are frequently identified in emergency situations, you can be ready to talk to your doctor about the matter at your next appointment if you're worried about your risk of stroke.

What you're capable of

Put down and be prepared to discuss the following if you would like to talk with your doctor about your risk of stroke:

Your stroke risk factors, like a family history of strokes,

A complete medical history that includes a list of all prescribed drugs and any vitamins or supplements you now take

Important personal details, like lifestyle choices and significant stressors

What symptoms you had and whether you believe you had a TIA

Any queries you may have

What to anticipate from your physician

In order to assess your risk factors, your doctor can advise you to undergo a number of tests. They should also advise you on how to get ready for the tests, such as fasting before having blood drawn to evaluate your blood sugar and cholesterol levels.

Exams and diagnosis

Your doctor may diagnose a transient ischemia attack (TIA) only on the basis of your medical history, without referring to any findings from a neurological or general physical examination, because TIAs are temporary. Your doctor may use the following information to help identify the cause of your TIA and evaluate your risk of stroke:

testing and physical evaluation. Your physician may perform a check for high blood pressure, high cholesterol, diabetes, and elevated homocysteine levels, which are risk factors for stroke.

In order to detect atherosclerosis, your doctor could also use a stethoscope to listen for a whooshing sound, or bruise, over your arteries. Alternatively, during an ophthalmoscope examination, your doctor may spot platelet or cholesterol particles (known as emboli) in the tiny blood vessels of your retina, which is located at the back of your eye.

carotid ultrasound imaging. A transducer, which resembles a wand, inserts high-frequency sound waves into your neck. Following the passage of sound waves through your tissue and back, your physician can examine images on a monitor to check for carotid artery constriction or clotting.

scanning for computed tomography (CT). Utilizing X-ray rays, a CT scan of your head creates a three-dimensional composite image of your brain.

scanning with computerized tomography angiography (CTA). The arteries in your neck and brain can also be noninvasively assessed using a head scan. Similar to a routine CT scan of the head, CTA scanning involves X-rays but may additionally require the injection of a contrast agent into a blood artery.

MRI stands for magnetic resonance imaging. This process can produce a composite three-dimensional image of your brain using a powerful magnetic field.

MRA stands for magnetic resonance imaging. This is a technique to assess the arteries in your brain and neck. It employs a powerful magnetic field, much like an MRI.

echocardiography. A transesophageal echocardiography (TEE) or transthoracic echocardiogram (TTE) may be performed by your physician. A transducer is a device that is moved across your chest during a TTE. An ultrasound image is produced when the transducer generates sound waves that bounce off various sections of your heart.

A flexible probe with an integrated transducer is inserted into your esophagus, the tube that runs from the back of your mouth to your stomach, during a transesophageal echocardiogram (TEE). It is possible to create more precise and crisp ultrasound images because your esophagus is situated right behind your heart. This makes certain objects, such blood clots, easier to identify that might not be apparent during a conventional echocardiogram examination.

Arteriography. This process provides an image of your brain's arteries that is not often visible with X-ray imaging. Typically in the groin, a small incision is made and a thin, flexible tube called a catheter is inserted by a radiologists.

Your major arteries are used to guide the catheter into your carotid or vertebral arteries. The radiologist will next inject a dye through the catheter to produce X-ray images of your brain's arteries. This process might be applied in certain circumstances.

MEDICATIONS AND SUBTLES

The aim of treatment, once your physician has identified the reason of your transient ischemic attack, is to rectify the abnormality and avoid a stroke. Your doctor may recommend surgery or a balloon technique (angioplasty) or prescribe medicine to lessen the likelihood for blood to clot, depending on the reason of your TIA.

Drugs

Several drugs are used by doctors to reduce the risk of stroke following a transient ischemic attack. The location, etiology, severity, and kind of TIA all influence the treatment that is chosen. There are two common medication categories that are prescribed:

anti-platelet medications. One of the circulating blood cell types, platelets, are less likely to clump together when you take these drugs. Sticky platelets that have been wounded in blood arteries start to coagulate, and blood plasma proteins finish the clotting process.

Aspirin is the anti-platelet drug that is most commonly used. The least priced treatment with the fewest possible side effects is aspirin. Aspirin can be substituted with the anti-platelet medication clopidogrel (Plavix).

To lessen blood clotting, your doctor can prescribe Aggrenox, a combination of low-dose aspirin and the anti-platelet medication dipyridamole. Aspirin and dipyridamole function somewhat differently.

anticoagulants. Heparin and warfarin (Coumadin, Jantoven) are two of these medications. Their impact is on clotting-system proteins rather than platelet activity. Warfarin is used over a longer period of time whereas heparin is used temporarily.

These medications need to be closely watched. Your doctor might recommend dabigatran (Pradaxa), a different kind of anticoagulant, if atrial fibrillation is evident.

Operation

Your doctor can recommend a carotid endarterectomy if your neck artery (carotid) is moderately or severely constricted. By removing atherosclerotic plaques from the carotid arteries, this prophylactic procedure stops another TIA or stroke from happening. The artery is opened by an incision, the plaques are taken out, and the artery is shut.

Angioplasty

A process known as carotid angioplasty, or stenting, is a possibility in some circumstances. In order to keep an artery open during this treatment, a thin wire tube called a stent is inserted into the obstructed artery and opened using a balloon-like device.

WAY OF LIFE AND DOMESTIC MEDICINE

The best ways to avoid a transient ischemic attack are to be aware of your risk factors and lead a healthy lifestyle. A healthy lifestyle includes routine check-ups with the doctor. Moreover:

Avoid smoking. Giving up smoking lowers your chance of having a stroke or TIA.

Limit your fat and cholesterol. Reducing your intake of fat and cholesterol, particularly trans and saturated fat, may help prevent the accumulation of plaque in your arteries.

Consume a lot of fruits and veggies. Nutrients like potassium, folate, and antioxidants found in these foods may help prevent TIAs and strokes.

Reduce your salt intake. Reducing your intake of salt and avoiding meals high in sodium can help lower your blood pressure if you have high blood pressure. Refusing salt may not stop hypertension, but for those who are susceptible to it, too much sodium can raise blood pressure.

Engage in regular exercise. One of the few natural strategies to lower your blood pressure without medication if you have high blood pressure is to exercise regularly.

Restrict your alcohol consumption. If you use alcohol at all, do it in moderation. For women, the suggested daily limit is one drink, and for men, it is two.

Sustain a healthy weight. Being overweight increases the risk of developing other conditions like diabetes, high blood pressure, and cardiovascular disease. Dietary and exercise-based weight loss can improve cholesterol levels and lower blood pressure.

Avoid using illegal drugs. Cocaine and other drugs are linked to a higher risk of transient ischemic attack (TIA) and stroke.

Manage your diabetes. Diabetes and hypertension can be controlled by diet, exercise, weight loss, and, if needed, medication.

THE END